The Race Isn't Given to the Swift…

Built for It!

Rolita Brownlee

The Race Isn't Given to the Swift…
Built for It!
Copyright © 2021 by Rolita Brownlee

Disclaimer: The following versions of the Bible may have been referenced: New International Version (NIV), King James Version (KJV), New Living Translation (NLT), English Standard Version (ESV), New King James Version (NKJV), New International Reader's Version (NIRV), Christian Standard Bible (CSB), Common English Bible (CEB), The Message (MSG)

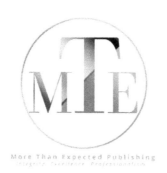

More Than Expected Publishing
Integrity Excellence Professionalism

MTE Publishing — mtepublishing.com

Dedication

My heavenly Father gets all the glory for this literary work; without Him, nothing in my life is possible! This devotional serves as commemorative work to my late father Walter D. Ward. I love you eternally. I extend my heartfelt love and gratitude to my parents, Madgerine and Darryl Bennett for your words of encouragement and support throughout my literary journey. To my loving and selfless daughter, Jaleah, thank you for always being my number one cheerleader! Lastly, this book is also dedicated to my family and friends, especially my sister in spirit, Dr. Gale Beasley, your friendship is an irreplaceable gift from God. Thank you for igniting the flame that started this process.

Literary Inspiration

Philippians 4:13 – I can do ALL things through Christ who strengthens me!

There is nothing more humbling than to receive an impartation from God when we least expect it! On December 26, 2019, during my alone time with God, this devotional was given to me. Upon completing this literary work, I sincerely understood that God Is My Strength (G.I.M.S.). In the eyes of men, many of us are not qualified to do what we do, but God created us and qualified us simultaneously for His purpose! Ecclesiastes 9:10 says, *Whatever your hand finds to do, do it with all your might, for in the realm of the dead, where you are going, there is neither working nor planning nor knowledge nor wisdom.*

Introduction

During Good Friday 1999, I accepted Jesus Christ as my personal Lord and Savior, through Billy Graham's online ministry. This was the MOST profound encounter of my life.

Prior to this experience, I did not have a clear understanding of who God really was… I did not have an intimate relationship with Him, *yet*! In the past, I'd <u>recited</u> the sinner's prayer however, I felt empty afterwards. Thankfully, on this very Good Friday, God opened my eyes. As I read the crucifixion story, I became overwhelmed with emotions, and tears began to stream down my face.

I sincerely understood that Jesus endured an agonizing death just for me! He loved me (and you) that much! At that moment, I <u>prayed</u> the sinner's prayer and felt every word within the core of my soul. I fell in love with Jesus Christ that day! I am forever grateful and honored to bear His name **CHRIST**IAN.

As a new believer, I desired to grow, so I spent [quality] time alone in His presence. God gave me an intercessor's heart. The Bible tells us that the prayers of the righteous availeth much. Consequently, my faith grew as I witnessed my prayers being answered. I learned to trust God in every situation despite the circumstances. A great deal of faith and trust in God was required for me to write this book. I tried my best to avoid the inevitable, but when God says *move*, we must lay aside our fears, doubts, excuses and trust Him *completely*.

It took me six months to draft this devotional. I am grateful that He used those close to me to ignite a fire of strength and determination to finish the work. Upon completion, I wept joyfully as I embraced and accepted the sovereignty of God.

Table of Contents

Chapter 1

Who is God to You?

1 John 4:16 - So we have come to know and to believe the love that God has for us. God is love, and whoever abides in love abides in God, and God abides in him.

Before responding to the question, take a moment to reflect. Think about how God is, what God is, why God is, where God is, and who God is [to you and for you]? Your response shouldn't be influenced by anything except your experiences and your relationship *with* God. These responses reveal who He is to YOU!

God is everything to me… He is ever-present in my life. He is the creator of the heavens and the earth. He is my Creator, who sculpted me and my life perfectly. He is my navigator; God guides my footsteps. He is the Prince of Peace; with God I remain in a state of serenity — no matter what. God deserves to be highly revered, so I worship Him in Spirit and in truth. This devotional is a personal love letter to Him that I want to share with the world. I know God loves everyone completely and uniquely. There is no greater love than the agape love He gives freely.

God is a spirit. Therefore, who He is, is evident in all creation. God is mysterious and unfathomable. He is above everything, yet God desires to commune intimately with us. His sovereignty is trustworthy because He is consistently loving and kind. He is the first person on my mind when I arise in the morning. Ultimately, God is the reason I can love and accept love… Matthew 22: 37-39 tells us, *Love the Lord your God with all your heart and with all your soul and with all your mind. This is the first and greatest commandment. And the second is like it: Love your neighbor as yourself.* So, it is with great anticipation that I crave intimacy with Him.

We were created to have an intimate relationship with God. Our relationship with Him should not be reduced to a two-hour Sunday service or one hour bible study. We must desire to seek Him, and God's word provides very simple instructions of how we can do this. James 4:8 reads, *Draw near to God and He will draw near to you.*

Why should we seek God?

1. Seeking God gives direction for our life, so we don't wander aimlessly. We have a purpose to fulfill, and God has already created the blueprints; it is up to us to follow His instructions for our lives.
   Scriptural Reference: Proverbs 3:5-6, *Trust in the Lord with all your heart, and do not lean on your own understanding. In all your ways acknowledge Him, and He will make straight your paths.*

2. Seeking God allows us to grow within our relationship with Him. We should not remain stagnate but continually evolve as God's chosen ones by applying His word in every aspect of our lives.
   Scriptural Reference: Proverbs 9:9-11, *Give instruction to a wise man, and he will be still wiser; teach a righteous man, and he will increase in learning. The fear of the LORD is the beginning of wisdom, and the knowledge of the Holy One is insight. For by me your days will be multiplied, and years will be added to your life.*

3. Seeking God, sets our priorities straight. He is more than life because without God our lives are hopeless and purposeless.
   Scriptural Reference: Matthew 5:6, *Blessed are those who hunger and thirst for righteousness.*

4. Seeking God produces the willingness to obey — ask, seek, knock. Our obedience moves God's hands on our behalf. He is the source of everything we need and desire.
   Scriptural Reference: Luke 11:9, *And I tell you, ask, and it will be given to you; seek, and you will find; knock, and it will be opened to you.*

5.   Seeking God renews our spirit and removes the clutter of sin, fear, doubt, bitterness, and unforgiveness from our lives. This allows us to see clearly and helps us see ourselves through the eyes of God.

Scriptural Reference: 2 Corinthians 4:16, *So we do not lose heart. Though our outer self is wasting away, our inner self is being renewed day by day.*

When to seek God:

Seek God in the morning, noon, or night — ANYTIME! Just enter into His presence with thanksgiving.

Scriptural Reference: 1 Chron. 16:11, *Seek the Lord and His strength; seek His presence continually.*

Where to seek God:

God is omnipresent, He is ALWAYS present!

Scriptural Reference: Jeremiah 29:13, *You will seek me and find me, when you seek me with all your heart.*

How to seek God:

1.   We seek God in spirit and in truth.

2.   Be still, quiet your thoughts and focus on The Creator.

3.   Listen to understand and respond by obeying His will.

Scriptural Reference: Luke 11:28, *But He said, "Blessed rather are those who hear the word of God and keep it."* Hebrews 11:6, *And without faith it is impossible to please Him, for whoever would draw near to God must believe that He exists and that He rewards those who seek Him.*

What does God require of us?

To simply LOVE and be a witness of who He is, we must:

1. Be still
2. Be patient
3. Be kind
4. Be the embodiment of His PURPOSE for our lives

What is the outcome when we seek God?

1. Personalized intimacy

2. Renewed mind and spirit

3. Reinforced faith

When we seek God, it is an open expression of our desire to align our actions with God's will, while we navigate through life. As we build an intimate relationship with our Creator, it is a display of our faith and trust in Him. Our obedience to God exemplifies our love for Him. Therefore, we understand and help others to see that God is our everything, undeniably!

Racing Thoughts — Take Time to Reflect

When you are in God's presence, embrace the silence so you can hear from His Holy Spirit. The Holy Spirit is a gift from God that guides you. Listen to the voice within, it will not steer you wrong; His sheep know His voice. Through the silence is peace, joy and understanding. Through the silence, He sharpens your sense of hearing. He wants you to experience His peace during your alone time. Sitting there in quietness allows you to renew your mind, spirit, and soul. Spending time alone, with God, starts your day off with a positive mindset because it is spirit led. Give God your undivided attention, which shows reverence for Him. Listen and hear from God!

What is God saying to you right now? Listen intently and respond accordingly.

_____

_____

_____

_____

_____

_____

_____

_____

_____

_____

_____

_____

_____

_____

_____

_____

_____

Chapter 2

The Race

Philippians 3:14 – I press on toward the goal to win the prize for which God has called me heavenward in Christ Jesus.

When most people think of a race, usually the first thought is how fast or swift we must be to *win*. As an avid runner, my ultimate goal is to maintain a steady yet swift pace. However, God's word tells us, the race is not given to the swift, but to the one who endures. So, I ask, whose race are you running today… your race, the world's race, or God's race? The world provides temporary gratification and leaves us empty. When we surrender our life to Christ, He becomes the center of our life, thus it is much easier to relinquish our need for control. This realization allows us to be martyrs for Christ. Trust me, this is an honor! Philippians 1:21 tells us, *For to me, to live is **Christ** and **to die** is **gain**.*

Although, it may appear that others have the upper hand because they finish the race before us, ultimately, we have the victory because Christ already determined that we are victors. The purpose of our race is not to run swiftly, but to walk with God as He guides us daily. Our entire life is a journey of self-discovery of who we are *in God*. Fortunately, as we accept this truth, we also understand the intricate connections we have to others as they complete their race, *too.* Ecclesiastes 9:11 says, *I returned, and saw under the sun, the race is not the swift, nor the battle to the strong, neither yet bread to the wise, nor yet riches to men of understanding, nor yet favor to men of skill; but time and chance happeneth to them all.*

Our Race is a Journey

Race and journey can be referenced simultaneously. As we follow the path that God has laid before us, our focus shouldn't be the finish line but the journey and resources we utilize along the way. As I write this book, I am currently prepping for my first natural bodybuilding competition in the figure division. I set fitness goals frequently and this competition is number three on my list. My focus has been the journey, not a race to get on stage. I am embracing every moment, which includes the valley lows and mountain tops. I am keeping God at the forefront. Every morning before I step foot in the gym; I happily bow in God's presence because our alone time is vital to my success. In His presence, I am transformed, rejuvenated, and strategically instructed… God gives me everything I need.

At times, our journey will be difficult because it is filled with lessons, hardships, and heartaches but God gives us peace. We can experience peace through the storms of life when we trust God completely. Philippians 4:6-7 says, *Do not worry about anything, but pray and ask God for everything you need, always giving thanks. And God's peace, which is so great we cannot understand it, will keep your hearts and minds in Christ Jesus.*

Preparing for the Journey Ahead: The Armor of God

To be effective in our spiritual journey we must equip ourselves with the whole Armor of God. The armor of God represents the defense we must take in our spiritual lives. The Bible tells us that we are fighting a war against Satan, who seeks to steal, kill, and destroy us. According to various online Christian study sites, we must be alert and put on God's armor, daily.

1.   **Belt of Truth**

The belt is vital to every soldier; it was used to hang battle tools. This belt also held the soldier's robe together. To the Christian soldier a belt of truth means that we are surrounded by honesty, truthfulness, integrity, and sincerity. Therefore, every part of our life is governed by truth.

The Lord knew our loins needed to be wrapped in truth. Regardless of the culture or time we live in, the Lord has seen all the paths we have taken and how they have hurt and derailed us. He knows we need truth.

Just as a belt is worn close to the body, we should hold God's truth close to us and allow it to surround us. When we remain in His Word, we can distinguish what is true from what is untrue. By remaining in His word, we will be fully equipped for spiritual battles that *will* come our way. Ephesians 6:14 says, *Stand firm then, with the belt of truth buckled around your waist.*

2.   Breastplate of Righteousness

The second piece of the armor of God that Paul discusses in Ephesians 6, is the breastplate of righteousness. In the armor of a Roman soldier, the breastplate served as protection for some of the most important organs of the body. Therefore, if a soldier did not wear his breastplate, he was vulnerable to an attack that could result in instant death. Righteousness means being made right. Sometimes scripture refers to righteousness that Christ gives us — His righteousness. It also refers to righteousness that God carries out through us. Revelation 19:8 says, *Fine linen, bright and clean, was given her to wear.* Fine linen stands for the righteous acts of God's holy people. Nevertheless, we need the complete righteousness of Christ, but also the continuing righteousness that comes as a response to God' gift. The enemy tempts us with all kinds of sinful entanglements, but righteousness protects our hearts. God's instructions are often viewed as killjoys or burdens. However, obedience to God protects your heart from being wounded.

3.   Gospel of Peace

As Christians, we are called to share the good news of Christ with others. Having our shoes fitted with the gospel of peace allows us to do this successfully. John 14:27 reads, *Peace I leave with you; my peace I give to you. I do not give to you as the world gives.*

Our shoes equip us to walk through rough areas. In the same way, having hope in Jesus helps us walk through the trials we face. John 16:33 says, *I have said these things to you, that in me you may have peace. In the world you will have tribulation. But take heart, I have overcome the world.*

Having confidence in Christ allows us to boldly proclaim His name. While we may face persecution in *this* life, we can rest in knowing the Savior of the world loves us and cares for us. Having our feet fitted with the shoes of the gospel of peace allows us to be ready to share the good news with others (at all times). As Christians, we should always be prepared, as we never know when an opportunity may arise to share love of Jesus with someone else. Ultimately, the shoes of peace equip us to fight for Christ in the spiritual battles we face.

4.   Shield of Faith

This is the fourth piece of armor Paul discusses in Ephesians 6. He tells us to take up the shield of faith in order to extinguish all the flaming arrows of the evil one. For a Roman soldier, a shield was used as another vital form of protection.

A Christian's shield of faith needs to be regularly dipped in the water of God's word to be replenished and fully functional. Romans 10:17 says, *Consequently, faith comes from hearing the message, and the message is heard through the word about Christ.*

Focus on God's track record, not on your circumstance.

5.   Helmet of Salvation

The helmet of salvation is another essential part of the armor of God. In the Roman army, the helmet served as protection for the head. It was a crucial piece of the armor, as an attack to the head could result in sudden death. Salvation comes the moment we place our trust in Jesus' death and resurrection as the payment for our sins. But salvation is also worked out through a lengthy process of sanctification. The helmet of salvation (like the breastplate of righteousness) rests on the work of Christ to save us. However, it also involves us as we journey with the Lord. The warzones of our mind is the primary place spiritual battles are fought. The Lord works His freeing truth to our advantage, while the enemy fights for strongholds to bind us. John 10:10 says, *The thief comes only to steal, kill, and destroy; I have come that they may have life, and have it more abundantly.*

6. Sword of the Spirit

The sixth piece of armor that Paul discusses in Ephesians 6, is the sword of the spirit, which represents God's Word. For a Roman soldier, the sword served as an offensive weapon against enemies. When sharpened, the sword could pierce through just about anything, making it a very dangerous tool.

To understand the connection between the sword and the Word of God, it is important to understand the power of God's word. Hebrews 4:12 says, *For the word of God is alive and active. Sharper than any double-edged sword, it penetrates even to dividing soul and spirit, joints and marrow; it judges the thoughts and attitudes of the heart.* Through the Word of God, we can clearly decipher between right and wrong. As a result, we can strive to live in a way that is free from sin. His word is the ultimate truth, and we find confidence in knowing it is our greatest weapon. If we are lacking in knowledge of the Word, we will struggle to fight against the enemy. However, those who seek God through his Word and abide by it will be blessed. John 5:24 says, *Very truly I tell you, whoever hears my word and believes Him who sent me has eternal life and will not be judged but has crossed over from death to life.* Sometimes, it is not easy to take up our swords and fight against the enemy. However, we are not called to do this by our own strength. When facing trials, we can find peace in knowing that God is on our side. Romans 8:31 reads, *What, then, shall we say in response to these things? If God is for us, who can be against us?*

When we are tempted, the most effective weapon that God has given to us as believers is the sword of the Spirit, which is the Word of God.

7. Praying in the Spirit

Ephesians 6:18 says, *And pray in the Spirit on all occasions with all kinds of prayers and requests. With this in mind, be alert and always keep on praying for all the Lord's people.* Romans 8:27 says, *And he who searches hearts knows what the mind of the Spirit is, because the Spirit intercedes for the saints according to the will of God.* Jude 1:20 says, *But you, beloved, building yourselves up in your most holy faith and praying in the Holy Spirit.*

God often gives me acronyms when I am studying His word:

For example, the word RACE:

R	Remain in His presence
A	Accept His word/will
C	Concise, His word is clear
E	Execute, His word — it's the plan for our life

R   Remain in His presence

How do you **prepare** for a race? As a sprinter, I took the leap of faith and set two fitness goals, to run long distance (a half and full marathon). I followed a set plan for both, which included conditioning, consistency, commitment, will power, patience, reading about the sport and most importantly keeping God at the forefront. My prayer was to stay injury free; God allowed me to do exactly that. Distance running is where I developed my alone time with God. Most people have on headsets, but God needed my full attention. In order to listen to God, you must be still, quiet your spirit, clear your mind and know that He is ever-present. Once you tune out everything else, you can hear clearly and allow God to direct your path.

A   Accept His word

When I made the decision to invite Christ into my life, I simply believed, confessed my sins, and accepted His word. *So, faith comes from hearing, and hearing through the word of*

Christ (Romans 10:17). Adhere to God's will and commandments, this is how we accept His will!

C   Concise — God's word is clear

Contrary to what anyone says, God's word is plain and clear. *He is not the author of confusion* (1 Corinthians 14:33). Therefore, we must eliminate unnecessary speech. Do not gossip or babble. We must remain focused in our conversation and speak on things that edify ourselves and the body of Christ.

E   Execute — God's word is the plan for our life

Being obedient and doing the will of God. *Blessed rather are those who hear the word of God and keep it* (Luke 11:28).

God also planted the word **PACE** in my spirit because He sets the pace for our journey:

P   Peace going down the path He has set before us
A   Attention to Him, Seek Him
C   Confidence in His word, this is faith
E   Enlightenment, understanding brings revelation

The race is not given to the fastest; they are overlooked because of pride, selfishness, and following their own philosophy in life. *Many are called but few are chosen* (Matthew 22:14).

Who are the chosen?

1.   Those who are Godly
2.   Those who are after God's heart
3.   Those who desire God
4.   Those who show humility
5.   Those who show empathy
6.   Those who are witnesses

7.   Those who seek God wholeheartedly

8.   Those who allow God's light to shine in their lives

9.   Those who are committed, consistent, and confess sins often

10.   Those whose characters are flawed but work to mirror Christ

Model your life after Christ. Jesus died on the cross that we may have life and life more abundantly. Be saturated with the word of God. The Bible is so much more than just a book; it is manna from heaven. It is where we study God's word and ask for understanding so we can apply it to our daily lives. Through God's word, our mind is transformed, and our hearts are purified. Open your heart and apply God's word daily; remain hopeful and faithful; and trust and obey Him.

Do not burden the Holy Spirit, this is a precious gift from above; respect Jesus' bloodshed by honoring Him with your lifestyle. And remember there is power in the spoken name of Jesus!

Alone time with God

1.   Each encounter is different; there is no set script.

2.   Allow the Holy Spirit to flow freely. Allow God to lead.

3.   Thirst after peace, joy, kindness, goodness, gentleness, faithfulness, patience, self-control, and love. These are the fruits of the Spirit.

4.   Make time, not excuses. Prioritize God in your life.

Psalm 121:12 tells us, I will lift up mine eyes unto the hills, from whence cometh my help. My help cometh from the Lord, which made heaven and earth.

Get on your knees and bow down before God (as a sign of surrender). What are you surrendering? You are surrendering your will for God's will. He is your Creator, your Peace, and your Guide. You should fear Him, love Him, exalt His name, and respect Him because He is our Abba Father.

You just need to believe and have faith that He died and rose again so that you may have eternal life. Be strengthened in your walk. Remember this scripture, *I can do all things through Christ who strengthens me* (Philippians 4:13).

How did Jesus gain strength while on Earth?

1. Retreated to His alone time with God. Seek God
2. Kept the lines of communication open
3. Recited scripture to encourage Himself
4. Remained faithful, despite persecution
5. He knew He was predestined for greatness

Commit to living a life that's pleasing to God. Even when things seem to go awry in your life, God did not make any promises that we would not experience storms. However, He did promise that He would never leave our side. Learn to lean on Him, trust Him, remain in HIS presence, seek Him daily, listen for His voice, and allow Him to guide your footsteps. Remember, your race is a journey, speed isn't the focus, but enduring until the end is the goal. Psalm 62:8, *Trust in Him at all times, you people pour out your hearts to him, for God is our refuge.*

While seeking God on your journey —Take time to reflect

God must come first in our lives! He is a jealous God. *Do not worship any other god, for the Lord, whose name is Jealous, is a jealous God* (Exodus 34:14). Honor God by giving Him your best first and not your least. He is waiting! Your intimate time with God should be the main priority of your daily routine, especially in the morning. Acknowledge Him as the one who is sovereign in your life. Prepare for your day and life by seeking God first. Allow God's will to be done in your life, purposely.

What are you doing to have deeper intimacy with God? Write your plan of action.

_____

_____

_____

_____

_____

_____

_____

_____

_____

_____

_____

_____

_____

_____

_____

_____

_____

_____

_____

Chapter 3

Be Still... Faithfully

Psalms 46:10 - Be still, and know that I am God.

When we still ourselves in God's presence it allows Him to make deposits into our spirit. I have learned to quiet my thoughts and understand that the silence allows me to hear God's voice and focus on His instructions. God will direct our path, light the way, and shine ever so brightly in our lives. When we are alone in God's presence, He restores our hope, faith, and renews our strength daily.

If you don't know how to meditate and focus on God; this is for you. First, we must step out of situations to view them from a sound perspective. Observe before responding. Don't be so quick to react in anger or judgment. Give the Holy Spirit a chance to guide you in your decision-making progress. Listen for direction concerning your life. Our journey is not meant to be swift, but purposeful. We must learn to move slowly, and more importantly, *be still!*

The practice of *being still* is **S.T.I.L.L.N.E.S.S.**: It is **S**ilence that leads to feeling **T**ranquil and **I**ntrospection while we **L**isten and **L**earn why God is a **N**ecessity. Fortunately, in **E**xercising our intentional focus on God we will be **S**atisfied and embrace God's **S**overeignty.

S	Silence
T	Tranquility
I	Isolation/ Introspection
L	Listen
L	Learn
N	Necessity of God
E	Exercise your senses (hearing, seeing through God's eyes)
S	Satisfy
S	Sovereignty

S   Silence

What does it mean to be _silent_ in God's presence? Simply put, it means to be quiet and listen to hear from God for direction concerning your life. You must quiet your thoughts, which allows you to F.O.C.U.S. and give God your undivided attention. I love my early morning alone time with God. The world is still asleep, it is so peaceful, and I am able to focus my attention on things above. It is my time to commune with God.

F   Free your mind of clutter (fear, anxiety, pride, guilt, boastfulness...) Release those things not of God and allow Him to fill your mind with His thoughts. Surrender your will and meditate on God's word.

O   Open your mind to the ways of God. Devote yourself to living a fruitful lifestyle, displaying the fruits of the spirit (love, peace, patience, gentleness, goodness, kindness, self-control, faithfulness and joy). When you open your mind, you allow God to deposit into your spirit His unchanging word. You are showing obedience, a willing spirit and have an expectation for what God has in store concerning your life.

C   Commit to a Christ-centered life because he lives in you! You represent to the world what a Christian looks like. Your life should be centered around Jesus Christ. He bridges the gap between man and God. Through His sacrificial death, we were made right before Him. We must acknowledge Christ in all that we do. His death was not in vain concerning our lives. We live to bring glory to His name.

U   Universe — God created it all! We were created with a purpose, yet a free will to live life as we choose. Make Godly choices. God is ultimately in control of it all. He knows how many hairs are on your head. He knows your end to your beginning. He knows your daily journey. This is His world, not man. Appreciate the beauty of the sunrise/sunset. How birds take flight. How mothers care for

23

their young and fathers protect their offspring. Do not get caught up in the day-to-day hustle and bustle of life. Rather, celebrate his creation as you focus and run the race that God has before you.

S   <u>Step into the newness</u> of Christ. Once you give your life to Christ, the old nature ceases to exist. Behold all things are new! Walk in your purpose! Allow Christ's light to shine ever so brightly in your life. Live a purposeful life, on purpose. Be kind to others despite how they treat you. Develop discipline to patience and self-control because the enemy will rise against you. Be bold and obedient! Do God's will, do not make excuses; mirror the life that Christ lived. Salvation brings newness, a new mindset; so, a man thinketh he does. Confess your sins often, and ask God for help and grace with your weakness.

Silence builds patience, which strengthens your character. But they that wait upon the Lord shall renew their strength; they shall mount up with wings as eagles; they shall run, and not be weary; and they shall walk and not faint. (Isaiah 40:31) It is in the silence where you are being transformed into what God has predestined for your life. You can only hear Him through the silence you create. Turn off the noise of the world. In the silence, God is teaching you to be patient; be still, be quiet and listen to what He is saying. God speaks through people and circumstances. Pay attention, be alert, allow the Holy Spirit to guide and lead you, daily.

T   Tranquility

The state of being peaceful and remaining composed even in the midst of adversity. *And the peace of God, which surpasses all understanding, will guard your hearts and your minds in Christ Jesus* (Philippians 4:7). Peace comes from God! In HIS presence, we lack nothing. It is during our time of intimacy with God that we are renewed and strengthened. The peace of God is unshakable. Therefore, we can remain still in the midst of chaos by:

1.   Remaining focused on God

2.   Understanding that God controls our destiny

3.   Believing God for His word to manifest

4.   Trusting God faithfully

I   Isolation & Introspection

Tune into the presence of God. He is always available to meet your needs. I have a standing daily appointment with God every morning around 4am. I set my alarm, the night before with great expectation of our morning encounters. As the alarm sounds, I awaken refreshed with excitement to hear from my Abba, Father. I fall to my knees by my bedside and begin to thank God for my many blessings as well as confess those things that would hinder my alone time. I bask in the presence of God and allow him to lead during this sacred time. James 4:8 says, *Draw near to God, and he will draw near to you. Cleanse your hands and purify your hearts, don't be double-minded.*

L   Listen

How do you listen to God? Clear your mind and tune into what the Holy Spirit is saying.

When you spend enough time seeking God, you become familiar with His voice. You are able to stay focused and listen with great intent regarding instructions on how to run your race:

- Be slow to anger
- Be slow to respond
- Be slow to react
- Be slow to cast judgement

This allows you to be gentle and to show love. Sometimes God does not want you to respond but to remain humble, which can be tough at times, trust me, I know. You develop patience when you listen. Our ears are the gateway to understanding; we must use them to listen. Therefore, when you hear the word of God, you will apply it to your life. *He that hath ears to hear; let him hear* (Matthew 11:15).

L   Learn

To have a godly mindset, you must spend time alone in his presence, saturated in his word to seek understanding, which gives you wisdom. I try my best to submerge myself in the word through my morning, afternoon, and evening devotions. Oftentimes, God confirms, throughout the day, what He spoke in my spirit during my 4am devotion. I find that spending time in His word better equips me for the day at hand. Psalm 119:11, *I have hidden your word in my heart that I might not sin against You.*

N   Necessity of God

Do not impress man but be faithful to God. The race is not given to the swift. The swift do not have time to listen and hear from God. They go at their own pace in life. You need to rely on God! Proverbs 3:5-6 tells us, *Trust in the Lord with all your heart and lean not on your own understanding; in all your ways submit to him, and he will make your paths straight.* Stillness is where you wait on the Lord for guidance and strength. It is where you take a pause to hear from God; so listen closely. Hear what He is telling you, be a doer of His word and hide it in your heart; do not sin against God! Here's how to prepare for the battle.

1.   Spend alone time with God
2.   Read God's word
3.   Apply God's word
4.   Be Still and you will know
5.   Listen to hear from God
6.   Communicate with God throughout the day

E   Exercise your senses (hearing, seeing through God's eyes)

Our thoughts are not His thoughts; our ways are not His ways. God is looking for obedience, faithfulness, fruits of the spirit displayed in your character, a willing heart. Again, the race is a lifelong journey — be prepared! Suit up for your race each day!

S   Satisfy

Only God can provide the soulful satisfaction we need. When we feel depleted, uncertain, lonely, or misguided; it is usually because we've sought people or things outside of God's will. Matthew 5:6 reads, *Blessed are those who hunger and thirst for righteousness, for they shall be satisfied.* When we allow God to satisfy us, He satisfies us in every capacity because it's what He promised. Therefore, we should intentionally reflect on and apply Matthew 6:33 to our lives, *"But **seek ye first the kingdom of God**, and his righteousness; and all these things shall be added unto you."*

So, embrace an attitude of reverence; and express it your daily life.

S   Sovereignty (God rules, God reigns)

God is present in every situation. He is our Creator, and He never desires to be separated from us. Sometimes God wants us to slow down and stop running the race because walking and being still are required at times. We are not waiting for God to catch up, but we are accepting His leading. God determines our pace, and it is perfect. So, just trust His sovereignty because God knows our story from beginning to end!

While You're Being Still — Faithfully, Take time to Reflect

God is faithful to us; this is the soul/sole reason we should trust Him. Our faith in God is never based on our abilities but His. Naturally, we tend to desire complete control, but God is the only one that knows everything about us... our beginning, middle, and end. Therefore, it is erroneous for us to believe that we can do a better job of planning our lives than God can. So, let's *be still...* faithfully!

If you find it difficult to be still, develop a strategy to create still time. Include meditation/prayer focus areas. Also, reflect on how you will trust God.

_____

_____

_____

_____

_____

_____

_____

_____

_____

_____

_____

_____

_____

_____

_____

_____

_____

_____

_____

Chapter 4

Fruits of the Spirit

Galatians 5:22-23 - But the fruit of the Spirit is love, joy, peace, patience, gentleness, goodness, kindness, self-control, and faithfulness.

During my alone time with God one morning, He spoke Galatians 5:22-23 in my spirit and instructed me to write it down and keep a copy on my nightstand, desk at work, and inside my vehicle. In doing so, each time I saw the scripture I was reminded that God was transforming my mindset.

I adhered to God's leading and dissected the word FRUIT

Fruit is a seed-bearing structure; a developing Christian's character is fruit. If our goal is to be Christ-like, then surely every trait developed within us should reflect His character.

Evaluate the fruit you produce in your life:

- Hate vs. Love

- Bitterness vs. Joy

- Stress vs. Peace

- Anxiety vs. Patience

- Cruelty vs. Kindness

- Selfishness vs. Selflessness

- Untrustworthy vs. Faithfulness

- Rudeness vs. Gentleness

- Anger vs. Self-Control

So, I say, walk by the Spirit, and you will not gratify the desires of the flesh. For the flesh desires what is contrary to the Spirit, and the Spirit what is contrary to the flesh. They are in conflict with each other, so that you are not to do whatever you want. But if you are led by the Spirit, you are not under the law. The act of the flesh are obvious: sexual immorality, impurity and debauchery; idolatry and witchcraft; hatred, discord, jealousy, fits of rage, selfish ambition, dissensions, factions and envy; drunkenness, orgies, and the like. I warn you, as I did before, that those who live like this will not inherit the kingdom of God (Galatians 5:16-21).

Fruits of the Spirit

Love

God is love, without love we don't have a connection to God. However, when we sincerely love people from our hearts, we allow them to experience God through us! So, if there is one thing, we should master — it is love! When we love, everything falls in place. Ask yourself daily; are you showing **love**?

Joy

Joy comes from within; it is a perspective of positivity and peace despite unfavorable circumstances.

Consider it all joy whenever you are faced with trials and tribulations because you know that the testing of your faith produces perseverance (James 1:23). Understand this; if people or things are the source of your joy, it is not of God. You will eventually experience emptiness, always wanting more and never fulfilled. God's joy brings contentment, despite the situation. Joy is a spiritual experience of having a personal relationship with God. Ask yourself, am I happy or joyful?

Peace

And the peace of God, which transcends all understanding, will guard your hearts and your minds in Christ Jesus (Philippians 4:7).

Peace starts in our mind, and it is a choice. I often experience peace first thing in the morning. In the quietness and stillness of the morning, I can focus on what really matters, my Creator. I make a conscious choice and take that peace with me throughout the day. Make the decision and give God full reign in your life — regardless of the circumstance!

P.E.A.C.E. is priceless

P	putting or placing
E	everything (all situations)
A	at a
C	calm
E	existence in our life

Patience

Be still in God's presence, which ultimately teaches you to be still regarding your daily walk and using discernment along the way. Wait on God; He will instruct, guide, lead you along your path; thereby fulfilling your purpose. Patience brings peace, which puts your mind at ease. When your mind is at ease, God can use you for His Kingdom. It causes you to smile often and encourage others to be in His service.

Kindness

Be kind and compassionate to one another, forgiving each other, just as in Christ God forgave you. (Ephesians 4:32). With the current climate of the world, we all could use Kindness. God created us to worship and love Him. We are to love our neighbors as we love ourselves. Kindness is shown in the simplest ways; it could be through a smile, hug, listening ear, financial blessing or humbling ourselves.

Goodness

Let no corrupt communication proceed out of your mouth, but that which is good to the use of edifying, that it may minister grace unto the hearers (Ephesians 4:29). Let us focus on building one another up instead of tearing each other down.

Faithfulness

The quality of being faithful, strict, thorough, and constant. God is calling for faithfulness. How can He enlarge our territory if we are not faithful in a few things? If you are faithful over the few, God can trust you with much. *For whoever has will be given more, and they will have an abundance. Whoever does not have, even what they have will be taken from them* (Matt. 25:29).

Gentleness

The quality of being kind, tender or mild-mannered; Showing humility and thankfulness towards God as well as polite, restrained, and compassionate behavior towards everyone else. Soft and calm and sweet to others. It allows us to explore all that is possible in ourselves, creativity to perform well and to work effectively with others:

- **Think** with gentleness
- **Answer** with gentleness
- **Respond** with gentleness

Self–Control

In character-testing situations, we must exercise self-control, because our emotions aren't always loving or rational. Self-control allows us to display the fruits of the spirit.

Experience peace amid chaos. If I may be candid here, this fruit was very challenging for me, but God has been ever so patient. I thank Him for His mercy, grace, and continued favor in allowing me to grow.

For the Spirit God gave us does not make us timid, but gives us power, love and self-control (2 Timothy 1:7).

While You're Planting, Growing, and Producing — Consider the Harvest.

Everything we do is ultimately a seed planted. Therefore, we should ensure that our actions align with the fruits of the spirit. Is this easy? Not all the time; however, when we align our actions with the Word of God, the outcome is *always* more than worth it. God desires to exceed our imaginations and expectations of Him. Surprisingly, God only requires that we follow His instructions… So, lets strive to be loving, peaceful, kind, gentle, mild-tempered, faithful, and good.

What are you planting? Reflect on your harvest, do your actions align with the fruits of the spirit?

_____

_____

_____

_____

_____

_____

_____

_____

_____

_____

_____

_____

_____

_____

_____

_____

_____

_____

_____

_____

_____

_____

_____

_____

_____

_____

_____

Chapter 5

You've Been Set Apart

When I look in the mirror, who do I see?

Someone who wants to do right

Someone who loves the Lord

Someone who asks, seeks and knocks during her alone time in His presence

Someone with a giving spirit

Someone who can be genuine and show compassion

Someone who exercises discernment

Someone whose spirit is willing, but flesh is definitely weak.

Someone who needs to do a better job proclaiming Christianity

Someone who does not always see the love of Christ within herself

Someone who needs to be consistent

Someone who needs to have a Christ-like mindset

Someone who needs to let go of the past and not worry about the future...

The above excerpt is from my journal entry on January 1, 2021. I look in the mirror daily and I conduct a personal checkup. I am patient with this woman looking back at me. I understand she is *still* growing and blossoming into the person God has called her to be. So, I thank God for her – because I understand the journey of becoming me is not a sprint. However, it is a series of marathons, and God gives me the strength to endure them all.

Matters of Heart

The heart is tricky because it doesn't evaluate life logically or spiritually, but emotionally. Fortunately, because God is so gracious, He assesses our commitment to Him based on what is revealed from our heart. God doesn't need us to tell Him anything, He wants us to openly communicate and be honest with Him. God can't help us if He doesn't hear us.

What are you telling God from your heart? *Above all else, guard your heart, for everything you do flows from it* (Proverbs 4:23).

Reconciliation

Reconciliation allows us to coexist in harmony. Christ reconciled us to Himself and gave us the ministry of reconciliation; that is, in Christ. God reconciled the world to Himself, not counting their trespasses against them, and entrusting to us the message of reconciliation. *Therefore, we are ambassadors for Christ, God making His appeal through us. We implore you on behalf of Christ, be reconciled to God.* (2 Corinthians 18-20).

Blessings

God promised to bless us beyond what we deserve. So, we must understand that God's favor on our lives isn't based on our love for God, but God's love for us! For this reason, God desires to see the love He has extended to us manifested in how we love others. This is how we grow and walk in our purpose. We are the epitome of God's blessings for all to see. Therefore, we were set apart to make a difference along this journey. Our lives are the blessing that someone else needs to encounter in order for God to bless them! *The Lord's blessing brings wealth, and He adds no trouble to it* (Proverbs 10:22.).

While you're embracing your uniqueness in God—Consider your difference

Every day we should reflect on how our lives make a difference. We should never seek to be like others, but be authentic as we let our light shine. When God created humankind, we were in the likeness of Him, not the exactness. Therefore, God gave each of us specialized talents, gifts, personalities, and appearances. We must embrace all of who we are to exude who God is! This is the way love is personified when we accept who we are in God and love others the way He loves us. It is in this manner we are set apart... We were fearfully and wonderfully created to differently exhibit the greatness of God!

How does your uniqueness contribute to your endurance?

_____

_____

_____

_____

_____

_____

_____

_____

_____

_____

_____

_____

_____

_____

_____

_____

_____

_____

Chapter 6

God Directs Our Path

Psalm 32:8 - I will instruct you and teach you in the way you should go; I will counsel you with my eye upon you.

When we follow God's path, our journey becomes sacred. Thankfully, grace is our portion, so perfection is not required. However, we must respect God and strive to live a godly lifestyle. Therefore, we should ask for a fresh new anointing each day; be intentional about prayer and about remaining in His presence throughout the day. Continually rely on God's strength and not our own. *It is in Him that we live, move and have our being* (Acts 17:28). Only faith in God will sustain us along our journey — not our strength, talent or resources.

God's Will

There is no better place for us to be than in the perfect will of God. Our obedience to God's plans proves our faith in Him. In reading Charles Stanley's book, *The Will of God*, I have shared the questions for the *Sevenfold test to confirm God's will.*

1. Are my actions consistent with the Word of God?
2. Is this a wise decision?
3. Can I honestly ask God to enable me to achieve this goal?
4. Do I have genuine peace about this path?
5. Is this decision appropriate for who I am as a follower of Christ?
6. Does this fit God's overall plan for my life?
7. Will this decision honor God?

God is our Creator; we are His children. He made each one of us with a purpose in mind, to live life and to live abundantly. Acquiring things or money provides temporary fulfillment. God fills our voids by giving us unconditional love. When we are thankful, obedient and allow God to lead; we are telling Him, "I will **go** where you tell me because I love you and trust you."

I am reminded of a powerful virtual bible study I attended at the onset of COVID-19. The lesson was taught by Dr. Gale Beasley, who gave this acronym for the word **GO: G- God, O- Ordained.** *You were set apart from the world; do not conform to the world. Be in it – NOT – of it. Be a warrior. Do not faint in well doing* (Galatians 6:9).

How do you allow God to direct your path?

Develop a routine of intimacy with God and follow His will for your life. God's directions for our lives are individually customized. Remain focused and stay on the path God prepared before you. Remove the distractions by identifying the things that compete for your attention (social media, TV, worry, people, etc.) Remember, the will of God provides protection, we should try our best not to deviate from it! So, be ready to run your race and be fully equipped with the armor of God.

God's Plans are Always Perfect — Our Plans Don't Compare to His

Naturally, we want to be in control because it allows us to have a sense of knowing. Unfortunately, we are not privy to the uncertainties of life so we cannot plan accordingly. However, if we place our trust in God, He will navigate our journey and ensure that our steps align with His plans. Our plans are mediocre when compared to the miraculous blueprints God has constructed. Therefore, if we allow Him to reign supreme in our lives, God will fulfill promises that we don't even know He has made to us! Now, if this fact doesn't make us trust the plans of God — nothing will!

Do you really believe God has orchestrated the BEST plans for your life? Reflect on your ability to place your life in God's hands, completely.

_____

_____

_____

_____

_____

_____

_____

_____

_____

_____

_____

_____

_____

_____

_____

_____

_____

_____

_____

_____

_____

_____

_____

_____

_____

_____

_____

Chapter 7

S.T.A.Y.

*Psalms 27:14 - Stay with God! Take heart. Don't quit. I'll say it again:
Stay with God.*

Society tells us that we have the right to stay or leave. In most instances, we weigh the pros and cons and decide what is best based on our feelings, resources, and logic. Fortunately, because we are God's children, He has removed the "guess-work" and provided a "fail-safe" navigation system within His word. When we invite Jesus into our life to S.T.A.Y., we eliminate the possibilities of failing and ensure that we will be victorious, no matter what!

S	Strengthened (Phil 4:13)
T	Trust (Proverbs 3:5-6)
A	Anointing (2 Corinthians 5:17)
Y	Yield to the Holy Spirit (Psalm 119:9-11)

Strengthened

I can do all things through Christ who strengthens me (Philippians 4:13). This is my favorite scripture because it reminds me that God is in control despite my circumstances. Through failed relationships, job loss, unforeseen disasters, uncertainty and death, God has given me the strength to endure every curve ball life has thrown. God has taught me, I am not promised tomorrow, so I choose not to fret about tomorrow's problems. Consequently, my strength is retained, restored, and renewed daily.

Trust

Trust in the Lord with all your heart and lean not on your own understanding; in all your ways submit to Him, and He will make your path straight (Proverbs 3:5-6). My sister in spirit, Dr. Gale Beasley, purchased several journals for me, because she knows me *for real*. One of the journal titles read, *"Trust in God, He Has a Great Plan for Your Life"*; glancing at the title, I am often reminded to Trust in God. By simply reading those words, the mood was set for me to have an indescribable encounter *with* God. I've come to understand that my trust in Him, is revealed in my obedience to Him. However, my disobedience will lead to unnecessary sacrifices and hardships. Trusting Him is much more beneficial than placing my trust in things, people, stuff or myself.

Anointing

And it is God who establishes us with you in Christ, and has anointed us (2 Corinthians 1:21). As a new believer in Christ 22 years ago, I was so anxious to be used by God! God blessed me with the gift of speaking in tongues, gave me an intercessor's heart, and the talent of praise dancing. I was anointed to do these things purposely. When God gave me the desire to challenge my physical abilities (marathons and bodybuilding), I did not foresee the creation of this journal and devotional, but He did! Therefore, I do not take God's anointing over my life for granted, but I cherish it and understand God's anointing is a gift from Him, and I gladly share it with others.

Yield

In your life together, think the way Christ Jesus thought. He was like God in every way, but he did not think that his being equal with God was something to use for his own benefit. (Philippians 2:5-7). I had to yield to God's will and not my own. I tried things my way, but they only worked temporarily. I have struggles daily, but it was my willingness to trust God that has caused elevation and blessings. So, we must yield to Him willfully. It is with our heart that we please God, not our works.

God is Never Forceful, We Choose to Accept His Invitation. Yielding to God is as Simple as saying, "Yes, Lord, I Trust You."

Saying, "yes" to God seems to be difficult for so many of us. Relinquishing our need to be the dictators of our lives allows God to be the divine navigator. We cannot expect our plans to be the BEST, because our plans could never exceed God's plans. When we yield to God's sovereignty for our lives, we place ourselves in a position to be champions. Therefore, we are not seeking to be ranked higher than others – but we yearn to be the spokesperson for God's divine will. We are champions for Christ! We must remember that in the eyes of many men, Christ was weak, but in the end, His endurance proved that He was more than a conqueror because He stayed on the cross.

How many times have you rejected God's will and went your way? Reflect on the benefits of yielding to God.

_____

_____

_____

_____

_____

_____

_____

_____

_____

_____

_____

_____

_____

_____

_____

_____

_____

A Call to the Race

Our journey with God, is a race that is designed to help us achieve our purpose. We must understand that our race will not mirror anyone else's race. Even if we are racing at the same time, our path may have an obstacle that only we have been strengthened to endure. So, lets promise God and ourselves, that no matter how difficult our race gets, we will endure until our purpose is achieved!

Isaiah 43:1-3 states: *Fear not, for I have redeemed you; I have called you by name, you are mine. When you pass through the waters, I will be with you; and through the rivers, they shall not overwhelm you; when you walk through fire you shall not be burned, and the flame shall not consume you. For I am the Lord your God, the Holy One of Israel, your Savior.*

May we commit to God to achieve our purpose and experience His provision faithfully. So, I invite you to pray the sinner's prayer and begin experiencing a life freely and more abundantly. Make this prayer personal:

God, I come to You broken. I know that I am a sinner, and I ask for Your forgiveness. I believe You died for my sins and rose from the dead. I turn from my self-pleasing ways and invite You into my heart and life. I want to trust and follow You as my Lord and Savior. Thank You for accepting me as I am. I look forward to growing into the person You created me to be. Lord, strengthen me to run this race (called life) with your stride and grace. In Your name I pray. Amen.

Submit all prayer requests to: www.rolitalbrownlee.com.

About the Author

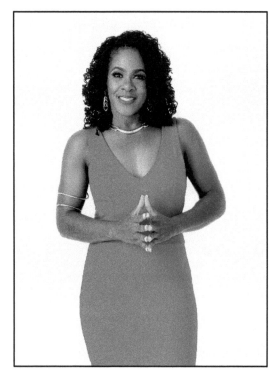

Undeniably, Rolita Brownlee is beautiful and strong. Most people would immediately attribute this to genetics and her intentional efforts to remain in optimal health. Nevertheless, while Rolita believes strength and beauty are some of our greatest attributes, we must never forget God is the source of it.

Rolita, affectionately known as Ro, is a certified personal trainer, competitive bodybuilder, and published author. She also has a professional background in accounting, insurance, compliance, and unclaimed property.

The Washington, DC native attended West State University and The Stenotype Institute of Orlando.

In 1999, Rolita founded a unique fitness brand and movement – God Is My Strength–G.I.M.S. The mission of G.I.M.S. is to empower fitness and kingdom ambassadors to exercise their mind, body, and spirit, while acknowledging that God is the source of their strength.

Rolita's passion for fitness started at very young age when her mother kept her active in cheerleading and dance. This led to a love for running, which started in high school. During that time, she was often compared to the likes of U.S. Olympic track and field legends, Florence Griffith Joyner and Valerie Brisco Hooks.

Rolita uses her fitness platform to propel her spiritual growth and to encourage others. It was during her prayer time that she was inspired to write her debut literary devotional, "The Race Isn't Given to the Swift...Built for It!" The inspirational journal inspires readers to get in the race [called life] and discover God's love, peace and freedom. The devotional is available everywhere books are sold, online (Amazon, Walmart, Books-A-Million and Barnes & Noble).

Rolita enjoys running marathons as well as preparing for bodybuilding competitions. In 2020, she placed in several divisions in her very first two shows. She won the OCB Chesapeake Classic Women's Figure (50+division) and the OCB Queen City Showdown Women's Figure (40+division). On October 8, 2021, Rolita fulfilled yet another fitness goal by becoming a NASM Certified Personal Trainer.

When Rolita isn't training for competitions or training clients, she is active in the community as well as her church. She is an intercessor and praise dancer. Rolita also enjoys traveling abroad, spending time with her daughter, parents, and friends. She also enjoys scrapbooking.

Rolita uses her Facebook pages (God Is My Strength – G.I.M.S. Rolita Brownlee), and her website (www.rolitalbrownlee.com) to solicit prayer requests and offer personal training services. She believes God created everyone with purpose and we all need His strength to fulfill it!

CPSIA information can be obtained
at www.ICGtesting.com
Printed in the USA
BVHW010918211221
624502BV00017B/336